Indian Summer

How to glow as an autumn rose

Clarissa Rodgers-Briskleigh

Contents

Introduction

Some of this book is in the first person and the reason for that is there isn't a lot of advice out there. When you look up post-menopausal energy, or even getting older, any photographs tend to be of well-tended men and women with beautifully-dressed silvery hair smiling gently at each other over cups of tea. In fact you could almost think that between the late forties and the safe harbour of the late seventies there is nothing but a void. Perhaps the youngest are fighting off the signs of age and the oldest have accelerated towards it, but there's a big gap re those who could and should be celebrating autumn.

Babyboomers are certainly challenging that image, as individuals, all over the place - the supermodel who can still rock a bikini (we hate her), the celebrity who had brilliantly successful cosmetic surgery, the athlete knocking spots off competitors twenty years younger - but there's still a perception they are exceptions to the rule and all the rest of us are home in front of the TV waiting patiently to reach the age of eighty and become interesting again, or at least stop exasperating our offspring. I've interacted with hundreds of others who weren't waiting quietly but there are, as yet, no true case studies of just how many "exceptions" there are. So rather than be grandiloquent in the third person and imply I spoke for thousands, I spoke as I found, some of it general, some specific. My teens were stuffed with angst, my twenties with marriage and a baby, my thirties with motherhood, a phased return to work and divorce, my forties with my career and my teenager. Rush, rush, *rush,* working too long hours, stressed out of my bracket, losing one parent, then the other, and ever rushing blindly headlong forward - I'd been so furiously working and paying a mortgage and being a fairly incompetent mum that I'd lost track of myself in the process. My daughter left for university and her own life, and my fiftieth birthday loomed up, then vanished behind me. Life begins at fifty? What a *crock.* I was old. I knew it, I accepted it, and I did vaguely wonder how I would fill in the time until I could retire and drop dead with a sigh of relief. Then my employer moved operations abroad and I was made redundant, in my mid-fifties.

We get one life. Most of it is spent responsibly answering to family, and you get to your fifties and run out of steam. More or less as expected, really.

And then - hello autumn - the sun starts shining, the weather warms up, and you are feeling good. In fact, you feel *great.* Chirpier than in *years.* Welcome to Indian Summer! So how do you use this unexpected boon – order a gross of cats, learn to knit, regret chances missed, tell yourself you are already too old, that you can't do things? Don't you *dare.*

The unexpected gift of energy and sunshine was probably designed by nature to be poured into a tribe of grandchildren. It is an absolutely *brilliant* age – not yet old, seasoned, mature, experienced – but for the first time in the history of our species, thanks to the Pill and planned parenthood, we don't have those tribes of grandchildren, and we don't always know what to do with all the energy suddenly on hand. That's why you bought this book.

You can skip the rest of this chapter because I've reached my anecdotage and have had to prune ruthlessly, but this one was left in because it is relevant. Thing is, there *are* times when you'll suddenly feel old. Just this spring I went abroad for a lively holiday and it really wasn't quite warm enough for sitting on the beach and in the pavement cafes late into the evening. I came back with a cold, was a bit stiff in the mornings, aching in various joints, even a bit deaf after a hellish double flight back. Indian summer was over, obviously, but I finally went sighing to the doctor to see if anything could be done at least about my hearing, because I was missing out on half the office gossip.

I'm nominating that woman for sainthood. She was a fresh-cheeked thirty-something, she could have glanced at my chart, recoiled, said *yes* you're old, what do you expect at your age? And I'd have crawled out of there and ordered a Zimmer frame.

Nonsense, she said instead. You flew with a head-cold, you're paying the price, and you should be as good as new in a few weeks.

So then I diffidently mentioned the stiffness and aching and she pushed and pulled at my legs and tied them into pretzels and said nope, no problems whatsoever, do a bit more exercise and the aches will go away.

More? I hadn't done *any* since getting back because I was feeling so ollllld. So I started again and although I'm not a slavish exerciser, if you really want to feel ancient and decrepit, do your usual full exercise routine after a few weeks break. But I felt better almost immediately. Well, stiff and aching in different places, but I remembered those places, they stop whinging if you keep going.

The sun came out again.

Taking stock

Some assumptions will have to be made, so let's make them early so we know where we stand. Assumption – you are basically in good health: the occasional twinge or grumble doesn't count. You're not in dire straits financially. You are post-menopausal. The last time your system changed so dramatically was in your teens, and this time round you've had just as many mood swings, spots, bursts of restless energy and slumps of sudden exhaustion. The after-effects of menopause are depressing - body-shape changes, drier skin, less biddable hair, and invisibility.

This section is called 'Taking Stock' because the vague idea is that you should recognise where you are and have a rough plan of what you want to do, and what you want to get from this book.

There's a lot of pressure on looking young these days - photo-shopped models, every flaw and blemish removed, are presented as the norm, actors and TV presenters insist on special filters being used on cameras. Every now and then cruel photos are splashed onto social media showing original publicity shots of celebrities, twenty or thirty years out of date, next to paparazzi pics which must make said celebrities want to eat their own livers in rage and frustration.

The message is loud and clear. If you don't look wonderful, you're a has-been.

The fact remains that we are statistically likely to live longer than our grandparents and parents. We have access to better food, and better health facilities, and age is not the absolute number it was. The clock in our head knows that, but the outer casket hasn't always stayed with the program, and the emphasis is on looking young.

This book can't make you look twenty years younger. What it is about is looking and feeling good. Not 'good for our age' - good, full stop. A *lot* of the book is about attitude, because people react to their first impression of you, and you react to their response. If they see you as tired and older, they will treat you as tired and older and you will *feel* tired and older. We want to be seen as interesting and worth getting to know, and age has little to do with that.

Part of the challenge of being where we are right now is that we can feel surplus to requirements. Empty nest syndrome, or the end of a long relationship – the death of a loved one who has needed nurturing for, sometimes, years - realizing we have probably gone as far in our careers as we are likely to get – mistakes made which we have to live with - sometimes merely that life wasn't the adventure we had expected it to be - are all downers.

Take hold, right now, and twist life back to where you want it to be. Your body, by the way, is 100% behind you on this. The human body is designed to live over a hundred years. Bits of us are capable of more—a healthy heart, for instance, can live much longer than the body it powers, even though young athletes can have heart attacks. We are potentially capable of being healthy and vigorous for a century. What we'll settle for is having the best Indian summer possible. Yesterday is over, tomorrow is in the wings, spending today in the sunshine is the day that matters.

We're called mature so I looked that up in my thesaurus:

  . *Fully developed powers of mind and body*

- *Complete in natural development*

- *Ripe*

- *Perfect (as in a plan maturing)*

- *Older than most (as in mature student)*

- *Grown up*

- *Fully fledged, developed, experienced, knowledgeable, sophisticated.*

Ah. Well, we aren't mature yet, then, although we're most of the way there.

Learn to walk

Oh, I'm not kidding. Try sitting in pavement cafes sipping coffee and watching the world going by, especially in holiday countries, and you'll spot it immediately. Moving well is very nearly a forgotten art, so it's the starting point.

You've heard the story that when Sean Connery auditioned for James Bond it wasn't an instant yes. One of the producers, though, was watching through the window when Connery left the building and remarked 'he moves like a panther'. The first, and for some the best, Bond had been cast.

There was a very funny mimic on the circuit not that long ago, *brilliant*. With just a few gestures, even just a well-timed glance, she kept transforming herself. At one point she went mid-step from a shambling teenager walking along engrossed in his iPhone, into a timid old woman. It was like that first time Michael Jackson did the moonwalk, just a few steps, and you were like *WHAT*? What *was* that? *Wow!*

It was quick, so quick, and then she had moved to the next imitation. She did it once more, later in the show. Such little things – dropping her head, losing the fluency of her stride, a shuffle. Lesson learned. The way you walk has instant impact, creates instant assumptions.

So your research starts in that pavement café. Put that wretched phone back in your handbag, life is far more interesting than anything on that dreary palm-sized screen. Sip your beverage of choice and watch people go by. You will see scuttlers, heads thrust forward, their feet scudding under them. Plodders, slumped and world-weary, never glancing at anything around them. Some women stalk like cranes in heels way too high for comfort. Some are relentless, feet well turned out, tramping endlessly through life. Most people are trudging along joylessly, getting from point A to point B, sometimes radiating sullen resentment that they have to walk at all. Some do walk like dancers, light on their feet, almost bouncing – mainly youngsters, but youngsters can also be dragging themselves along.

If you are lucky, you will see someone walking with their head high, their shoulders relaxed and moving nicely, stepping out and looking both relaxed and purposeful. That's an ageless walk, and it looks great. It is also good for you – less tiring than trudging, and carries a ton of benefits. Medically speaking, to walk tall, your head high, your neck long, your shoulders relaxed and open, means you are getting maximum oxygen into your lungs. Your feet are second only to your heart as efficient pumps, so walking gets your blood surging round your body, zooming through the heart, picking up oxygen and delivering it to every cell and molecule.

Add a tiny bounce to your step and it is a *look-at-me* walk, a celebration of being alive. All that extra oxygen whizzing around, you feel better, brighter, happier, and it *shows*.

Borrow a neighbour's dog, if you don't have one of your own, and practice while the dog distracts any spectators. Maybe working your shoulders with every step (the confident woman) or swaying your hips (the sex-pot), or simply walking so straight you are very nearly leaning backwards (the maypole) – well, along the way you'll be learning to walk for pleasure, your posture will improve, and while you don't need to go alarmingly far or fast it's a great way of ending your work day and starting the evening ahead. Going for a walk, with or without a dog, lets you hit your stride, reminds you how you should walk at all times. Which is as good a cue as any to mention the pet question.

Pets - yes or no?

There are pros and there are cons and it comes down to making the best decision for you. Even if you've always owned pets, you may choose to travel more in future, and then *you're* worried about *them*, and *they're* worried every time the suitcase appears, and it isn't ideal. If you've never owned a pet, don't rush into what is a pretty big responsibility and can be quite expensive, not to mention ultimately heart-breaking. A dog will make you go for walks, but that's not as much fun in the dark and cold of winter as it is on balmy summer evenings. Both dogs and cats will welcome you home (and escort you to the kitchen) with heartfelt delight. Puppies and kittens are hard work and can grow up into a pet you didn't expect or want. Rescue dogs and cats can need love and patience (a lot of love, and a lot of patience) to settle completely. It is a very personal decision, and it has to feel right, because mistakes are at least as traumatic for the unsuccessful pet as they are for you. I've lived with, and I've lived without. I said with the last dog, never again. My current dog is also a rescue dog, walks me all over town, and is invited along with me by hosts who don't want me to leave early. Sometimes you will have to cut short social engagements because you have to leave early. Going on holiday without them is a kennel-sorting mission. If you don't want a pet, don't have one, but do keep up the walking.

Posture

Back in the day our grandparents had to walk around with books on their heads but, perhaps because standing rigidly with locked knees in best military style, or sitting bolt upright with a hollowed back, isn't good for us, the baby got thrown out with the bathwater and posture is neglected. Poor posture isn't good for you either. Slouching cramps your lungs and twists your frame, and drooping slack-hipped, all weight on one leg, is not remotely good for your spine.

Imagine instead being lifted, your head in a gentle but firm clamp, and the rest of your body aligning itself from the neck down. Try to keep to *that* alignment, without strain, all your muscles comfortably supporting your skeleton.

That is of course directly related to the Alexander technique, which boils down to re-learning how to stand, sit, and, yes, walk. It is utterly simple. It is also so important it should be taught in schools, to become a lifelong habit.

If you have a desk job, make sure you sit properly, not hunched over. If you are leaning forward to peer, by the way, do you need glasses, or to update your present specs? Get up frequently and move around, always walking as though those 007 producers are looking for the next Bond girl.

Lower yourself gracefully when you sit, and fully into the chair, so the back supports you properly. Get into the habit of rising and sitting without heaving yourself around with your arms – use your core. Leave grunting and *oof* noises to tennis players. Twenty years before you need the sound effects – if ever.

Quickly skimming the basics

Eyes

That mention of spectacles, above – <u>get your eyes checked</u> if you are getting headaches, peering, or finding that your eyesight is changing, because it does, surprisingly often, in our autumn years. There are eye exercises you can do if you are determined not to go into specs (including the excellent Bates Method, which you can check out on line) or there is laser surgery.

The worst is of course labels on small bottles. Could we really ever read print that tiny? Get some magnifying glasses and keep one in every room of the home to avoid the frustration of straining to read something it takes you several minutes to realize is in another language anyway.

<u>Invest in good sunglasses</u> – you shouldn't have to narrow your eyes in glare at all, if your shades are good. Lovely as sun is, it can damage your eyes disastrously. Protect them. There are front-and-sides black-out pairs which can also go on over regular glasses and if you

can feel your eyes relaxing with relief when you put the hideous things on, *that's* priceless.

All pharmacies sell tiny expensive bottles of eye drops but all good pharmacies also sell fairly large bottles of <u>saline-based eye wash</u>, usually with an eye bath included. Blinking into an eyebath stings like the dickens if your eyes are very scratchy, and leaves you feeling like you had a good weep but when that passes, *bliss.* It does wonders for the whites of your eyes, too.

Teeth

The long-term benefits of <u>dentistry</u> really start paying off around this age. Good teeth are luck of the genetic draw, but well-cared-for teeth do last longer and look better. Missing teeth were cute when you were eight, not so much now. If your teeth are abandoning ship, bite the bullet and get good dentures or, if you can afford them, implants. This isn't just about looks - chewing your food properly makes for good digestion, and good digestion is *essential* for good health.

Even healthy teeth yellow with age, hardly surprising with everything you've thrown at them over the decades. Professional whitening or veneers cost a bomb but there are some quick saves in the 'quick fix' section for special events.

Hearing

The first time you notice you are missing things people are saying, it is worth getting your ears checked in case they need a simple old-fashioned syringing. Hearing is another genetic lucky dip, not helped by all those raves we went to in the Seventies. For sure the time will come when we'll be grumpy about the fact everyone mumbles and no-one can talk properly any more, but you may not know that exercise (no, *seriously*) can improve your hearing, especially yoga.

Mental exercises – crosswords, Sudoku, card games – and cutting down deadening noise – help hearing as much as they help mental agility. Constant noise is counter-productive. Listen when there is something you want to hear, and stop the sound when there isn't. Don't have the TV on permanently in the background. The current trend of music blaring into your ears through headphones or ear-plugs while exercising or commuting is not actually a good idea. Stress is also a factor in hearing loss – there's a proven link between stress and increasing deafness. There's a whole separate section on stress in the Fears chapter.

Skin

Your skin is the biggest organ in your body, and the older we get, the more of it we cover, but out of sight shouldn't be out of mind. Sun damage is a bit of a buzz word these days. On one hand, sunlight is vital to our health, a priceless source of Vitamin D. On the other hand, no-one, no matter their colour, can assume their skin needs no assistance - as with any vitamin, we can overdose. The lighter your skin, the more protection you need. If you are going on holiday, or spending more time in the sun than usual, use at least a Factor 15 and moisturise generously every day. Lightly-tanned healthy skin is way more attractive than the battered leather suitcase look. A *lot* of this book is about everything in moderation.

We're raising a whole generation of kids who will have bone problems because we have blocked their Vitamin D by plastering them in Factor 50+ – moderation, again. Enjoy it, don't bake in it. And help, don't use a sunbed, ever! That's about as far from moderation as it is possible to get.

Changes

You know not to ignore changes to moles, your digestive system, or anything you might put down to inevitable aging. In fact most things that happen are gradual and some may be genuine wear and tear, some could be easily corrected, and some are problems that should be nipped promptly in the bud.

There's a balance between worrying about every new symptom versus ignoring warning signs, and there's no denying luck does play a part. Our bodies have been changing since the minute of conception, mostly unnoticed, but we've reached the age of worrying. Read the Fears section before you brood over every tiny change. Often it is a simple problem, easily corrected, and you wasted any of your Indian summer worrying over *that*? You deserve better.

Good advice
first

There's some healthy advice and some serious topics coming up but this chapter covers the things you should absorb even if you give up reading when it gets serious. Some of them are obvious, some are reminders of what should be obvious. It's all about resetting attitude.

Enjoy your appearance. I've said before this can be an oddly invisible age, it's easy to slip into thinking no-one is looking so why bother except for special occasions? Actually more people are looking than you realize. Ignore the sillier fashion trends, but keep your own sense of style. It's part of who you are. Do your exercise, eat well, get your sleep. Keep yourself in good shape. Your Indian summer will be the longer for it.

Everything in your wardrobe should be in a colour and style that flatters you. Work out what you like best, and from now on buy clever, so everything you buy works with the favourites you own already. Hard dramatic colours can be teamed with softer pastels.

Scarves are fashionable, yay, that means tons of options out there! Good shoes are a must—good looking, and well-fitted. You're going to be walking a lot from now on.

Sing as loudly as you can, whenever you can. If you haven't done it for a while, the creaky croak may be a shock, all the more reason to sing more. In the shower, in the car, or join a local singing group. Fantastic breathing exercise and it will keep your speaking voice strong and vigorous for the rest of your life.

Always keep love alive. Love life, love your family, love your friends, love your neighbours. If you've been offended by someone – forgive them. If you've offended someone – apologise. Don't drag resentment with you. One thing we should have learned by now, it doesn't *matter* who was right. I can't remember who it was said that holding a grudge is like taking poison and expecting the other person to die, but it's true. Forgive, forget, and move on with your life.

We're at the age of change in our social interaction. Old friends move away, following their own dreams of living elsewhere, or are lost to you, and the thought of replacing a thirty-year friendship with someone new is, *yes*, daunting. Don't go grimly searching for new friends. Instead, find new things to interest you. In the process you'll meet others who share at least one of your interests. Friendships are like weeds, they grow in the most unexpected places.

If you hold strong beliefs, enjoy them, but don't waste your time trying to convince others. Live true to your beliefs, and respect the rights of others to theirs.

Do crosswords, and mental agility tests like Sudoku. Play cards, even solitaire. Bridge players seem to keep mental acuity longer than anyone else. Board games like backgammon, chess, and draughts, will stretch your brain. For that matter, any game that requires concentration and logic is good for you, and thanks to the internet you can pit yourself against players all over the world.

Learn to say no to invitations which don't interest you at all, and seek out activities which do. Include people who make you feel good, and exclude people who don't, even if you have known them for a very long time.

If you use social media (Facebook, Twitter, etc.) don't follow every link that presents itself. Story-shopping is accelerating mental confusion and reducing the ability of everyone, all ages, to concentrate. Do you really want to know, or are you just bored? Reduce your time on social media for the same reason.

Re-discover reading for pleasure. There are millions of novels out there, join a book-club or re-read old favourites to get back into it if you no longer read much. Reading is relaxing, but also excellent for engaging concentration. Cosy whodunits are ideal light entertainment as they reward concentration if you can solve the mystery before the end.

Fears

It's a given that by the time you're reading this either you've had a couple of health glitches, or friends have, or family. One result is that you've probably been consciously improving your general condition with a little judicious exercise, slightly more cautious diet.

So here we are, feeling better than in years, any offspring are for the most part now independent, the fierce competition of the workplace is less urgent: we've risen as far up the corporate ladder as we are likely to go. Time to ease back a little, and enjoy this unexpected Indian summer, right?

For some reason, no. Things are too good, we can't get used to that, so we turn this wonderful golden time into fears. We *could* get sick, so every symptom plunges us into gloom. We *could* lose our jobs, so we stress ourselves into getting sick (whoops, double whammy). We could lose friends, even people we love, and we start distancing ourselves in preparation. We've seen our parents get very elderly, or, worse, we've now reached the age they were when they died. Perhaps we're already older than they were when they died, so we feel we're on borrowed time.

And just yesterday you completely forgot where you put your handbag and you found it in the fridge and oh help Alzheimer's is beckoning.

And what the *hell* is this lump, how long has that been there?

Part of the 'mature and experienced' price tag is that we've seen a lot, and heard a lot of alarming stories. We weave disasters in our heads, and bingo, stress.

Stress is in fact essential to healthy living. Without challenges and pressures we would lead very dull and sedentary lives, and perhaps that's why, at a time we should be learning to relax, we manufacture threats.

The body copes very well, as a general rule, and being challenged actually makes you feel invigorated and purposeful. That's a physical reaction - stress triggers hormones designed to help you cope. Unreasonable stress, however, triggers the fight-or-flight emergency reactions. They flood your system, ready to haul muscles into extraordinary action, deal with the crisis, but there's no actual crisis and they can't burn off. Instead they accumulate, making you shaky, tense, and ultimately affecting your sleep, and that affects your health. Once your health is wobbling, you are actually creating the conditions you were stressing about. What's round and bites? A vicious circle.

Without awareness, you would unthinkingly carry a large heavy box downstairs, overbalance, go down the staircase like a human slinky, and the large heavy box lands on your head. Ouch.

With healthy awareness, you would go down cautiously sideways, aware you could overbalance, but with a plan in mind – drop the box and grab the stair-rail.

Unhealthy awareness would make you too scared to attempt to move the box, and you'd sit on the top step weeping with frustration at your helplessness, then go to bed with a raging headache and wake up heavy-eyed, unrested, and close to hysteria that you have to face these problems and it's *not fair* and you *can't cope*.

If you can see that box as a positive challenge, you trigger the right hormones to help you deal with it. Telling yourself you can't cope is not going to help. You can find a way to cope. That box, that job, that debt, those health fears – not one of them, not *ONE*, is helped by negativity.

Self-imposed stress is the unkindest thing you can do to yourself. Gloominess, martyrdom, feeling imposed upon, *why*? But if you insist, then go the whole hog. Find a pair of shoes which pinch and make you hobble, dig out an outfit which is a bit too tight and horribly uncomfortable, screw your face into a mask of patient suffering, and wallow in your misery. Then, for pity's sake, laugh at yourself and stop it.

Fears shrink into perspective with the right mental attitude. Life is 10% what happens to us and 90% how we react to it.[1]

Today, tomorrow, and for the rest of your life, remind yourself there are two things you should never automatically say again – *I can't*, and *I'm too old*. You probably can, and you probably aren't. You are mature, mellowed, experienced, and no matter what situation you find yourself in, you *can* cope. If you really want to do it, there's always a solution.

---

1. (attributed to a couple of people, but probably Charles R Swin-
   doll)

Chronic stress / depression

Sometimes the fears aren't imaginary, and reality becomes a little too real for comfort. Chronic stress, caused by an ongoing situation, is genuinely damaging. Managing it, or its dark cousin depression, is quite literally vital – they destroy sparkle, and put life itself at high risk. When it is a health issue, especially something long-term, mental attitude is a game changer. We all know about the denial, anger, bargaining, depression, acceptance, stages. Acceptance is one thing, resignation another. Adapt and seek the sun again.

The worst is self-induced - looking back in anger, in regret, even in anguish. NO. The past cannot be changed, the only thing we can change is the way we view it. Whether it happened to you, or whether you brought it on yourself, even innocently, you survived. Good judgement comes from experience. Experience comes from bad judgement. Letting yourself be warped by the past into chronic stress and depression is bad judgement, tantamount to locking yourself into a cycle of misery and throwing away the key.

Other triggers can be work-related stress, the terminal illness of a loved one, serious illness or trauma, amongst others, but once it has a grip you will need to seek professional help, because you will not be able to bounce out of this one unaided. There *are* a few things you can do to help yourself, because any part of your life spent on antidepressants is time lost forever. The more positively you work towards healthy mental balance, the less time you will lose.

One really good piece of advice from the experts is to shut down all outside sources of tension. Stop watching the news – headlines on the car radio is enough, if you feel you have to know. The media seems set on whipping us into a state of helpless rage or impotent distress, don't play that game. You've heard this quoted before: time to adopt it. "Grant me the serenity to accept what I cannot change, courage to change the things I can, and the wisdom to know the difference."

The *main* coping mechanism is quite simply sleep – both stress and depression hit you where it hurts, affecting your ability to rest and recuperate for the next grinding day. Anyone who has stared into three a.m., their thoughts racing as fruitlessly as a hamster on a wheel, knows how debilitating that becomes, night after night.

Natural sleep is the best, and the hardest to achieve. Exercise does help and even if you are bedridden, temporarily or otherwise, if you *think* your way through an exercise workout, your brain sends the same messages and the muscles tauten, relax, and tauten again. Not, obviously, as much, but there is a health-improving reaction, even some of the exercise buzz.

One bit of bright chirpy *infuriating* therapist advice is to go out socially. When you are living in the grey, nothing could be less appealing. Oh, it's true enough, but you cannot go from grey to gaiety just because some numpty says you should. Escaping the grey is hard, even if you are actively trying, even if the original source of the stress or depression has gone. It's a process, one tiny step at a time – and if you can make it a dance step, all the better. Bouncy happy music from bouncy happy times while you do some cleaning, both are oddly therapeutic. Housework is, this once, better than exercise, because the results are visually satisfying, and dancing through it will tire you nicely. Tiring yourself out will help you sleep. Sleeping will help you cope. When you are coping, you are tackling the road back to happy. Baby steps count.

A good night is the start to a good day

So – sleeping well is key to fighting off fears, stress and depression, and essential to good health. Well and good, but you may be finding around now that your sleep patterns are in flux. Just because you usually like to go to bed at ten, don't automatically go to bed at ten if you aren't sleepy, because you risk lying sleepless and starting to panic about it. At the same time, don't think there must be a problem if you are tired hours earlier than usual. Flux.

Many people hitting this interesting age do find that sleep is suddenly becoming elusive. They battle to doze off, wake in the early hours of the morning, or feel unrested when they get up. This can be either because they're ignoring the sleep patterns their body currently wants, or because there's some stress they haven't shaken off yet.

We don't actually need as much sleep as we take. Try not to fret about being the *only* person awake in the *world* when it happens. Doze and daydream and relax your limbs, and the occasional night will do no lasting harm. A glass of warm milk, or a Bach remedy such as Rescue Sleep, can do the trick at three in the morning for the occasional night when you realize at three in the morning that you aren't going to get back there naturally.

It's when it becomes the rule rather than the exception, when every night you start to tense up because you're afraid you won't sleep, and then you don't, that it is becoming chronic, and chronic sleeplessness is a bloody nuisance.

Sleeping pills really aren't ideal, try some of the options first. A rambling walk before bedtime. Chamomile tea and reading for ten minutes in bed. St John's Wort is good for chronic sleeplessness, but has to be taken over time to build up a cumulative effect. (It can counter-act with other medication, check with your GP if you are already on meds.) C-oil may need a little jiggling with the dosage before it delivers good nights with no heavy head the next day.

Breaking the cycle of bad nights is important. Sleep is becoming such a widespread issue that there are sleep clinics and experts in every direction. Not to be cynical, but since they make their living from sleeplessness, results can take a while. Try eating a small amount later, or a larger meal than your usual, earlier in the afternoon or evening. Don't have caffeine at all from noon onwards. If nothing works and you are starting to panic about your relentless inability to sleep, okay, you need to take more drastic action.

Taking sleeping pills as a habit, not good. Taking half a pill every now and then to break a cycle can really help. Even a tablespoon of cough medicine (of the *do not operate heavy machinery* type) can work a treat - after three bad nights, sleep is often coyly waiting to be beckoned. Alcohol, on the other hand, never a good idea. Good sex is unbeatable for a good night's sleep but sadly not always an option.

There are sleep whisperer recordings on YouTube but it can be unsettling, not relaxing, to be whispered to by a stranger. However, nothing stopping you making your own private YouTube recordings, murmuring quietly to yourself. Listening is instinctive, and overrides churning thoughts and since they're your own recordings they'll bore you to sleep nicely. Another way to banish churning thoughts is to get up, go to another room, and write down key phrases, promising yourself you'll sort them the next day. Equally if you are woken by pain or discomfort, get up and go write that down, then you can follow up the next day whether your physical symptoms have any suitable fixes.

Bottom line, sleep is natural to us and if there are no physical reasons we can't sleep, then we have unresolved issues, even if we don't realize it. Changing a habit can disarm an unsuspected trigger and approaching solutions calmly and methodically, knowing one of them will work, nearly always does the trick.

Exercise

Exercise is good for hearing, skin, appearance, posture, sleep, and quality of life, yet let's start with a warning. Not too much. Everything in moderation.

It's a temptation, when you are getting to an age where you are afraid of stiffening up or losing flexibility, to take on more and more exercise to turn back the clock. Like everything else, too much is counter-productive, straining or damaging joints and muscles. If you haven't done any for years, the mere word conjures up flushed faces, aching muscles and abruptly feeling very old and tottery indeed.

Without any exercise, your muscles lose tone, your skin starts to sag, you lose stamina, and energy and strength dwindle. This isn't about getting in training for the Olympics. This is about sprinting for a train without getting spots dancing in front of your eyes, or even just about touching your toes, although frankly it's been said if that was so important they should be on our knees.

Normal life counts - walking, gardening, housework, all good, especially if you add a musical soundtrack from the seventies, and bounce. Turn normal life into a workout, take the stairs instead of the lift, sweep the carpets instead of always using the vacuum cleaner, even a manual mower on the lawn instead of the power one - it mounts up. Walk to the post-box, don't take the car. You could do a lot worse than get a proper sit-up bicycle (one where you can put a basket on the handlebars) and pedal to the shops.

Life is filled with exercise breaks. While waiting for your bath to fill, swing your arms, do some knee-bends, twist your torso from side to side. Remember '*I must I must increase my bust, the more the better to fill my sweater*? *Very* good for firming up the bust-line and avoiding a future of tucking your boobs into your waistband. Pull gargoyle faces while you're doing your simple exercises. It isn't a workout, but it quickens your blood and feels surprisingly good.

Caught in a traffic jam and going nowhere? Play the piano on the steering wheel, open and close your fists, rotate your wrists. Work on your pelvic floor – tuck, release, tuck, release, and kept it up until the traffic starts moving again.

When exercise makes you breathless, it's all about emptying the lungs ready for the next breath. Don't suck in air when you are breathless, huff it out. There are breathing exercises you can do, but don't go crazy on them, I've recently heard of two people with COPD who had never smoked in their lives. One was a singer and the other played the bagpipes. Goes back to what we know already – everything in moderation.

Ten minutes of stretching every day, holding each position for ten seconds and not hurrying generally, will improve your flexibility dramatically. Simple yoga stretches are the best for these.

Roll your head gently, and look over each shoulder, about twenty times a day. It not only keeps your neck flexible, it stops it from thickening.

Your body shape is changing right now, and the chances are you will lose weight, especially if you switch your eating habits as suggested in the diet chapter. Exercise will stop you getting saggy and flabby as the fat melts away. Accept that perfection won't be happening, but target the bits that matter most to you – like adding shaker weights to actual exercise routines to get rid of bingo wings.

As for the type of exercise – maybe find an enjoyable dance routine lasting fifteen to twenty minutes, online or on a DVD, and set yourself to do it several times a week. You'll be stopping a few times to pant and strip off another piece of clothing, tomato-red and breathless, in the beginning. The stretches at the end are the best feeling in the world and bonus, sort out any back problems. ANY regular exercise – swimming several times a week, joining a yoga or pilates class, meeting up with friends to walk further than you would alone, tennis, golf, all good, pick the ones that feel okay because that will be what you enjoy and stick to.

Take a comfortably hot bath following a big workout (even a strenuous gardening session) to improve circulation and ease off any residual soreness.

Skip this paragraph if you're coy about sex. Thing is, happy sex is the most natural way in the world of boosting your heart-rate, getting your adrenalin jumping, and the closeness of a physical relationship, even if neither are you are sexual athletes, is priceless. If you do have someone, and aren't making the most of that priceless resource, what a waste. It isn't about swinging from chandeliers and strutting around in the nude looking magnificent because yup, that ship *has* probably sailed. You'd be lucky indeed to be burning off significant calories between the sheets - it's more about sharing your body with somebody else, and the awareness that brings. And burning off a few calories. An astonishing number of couples are finding that sex after menopause is in fact the best it has ever been. Woo your partner as much as you would woo a new person in your life, because the benefits for you both are lifelong - ask those bright-eyed rosy-cheeked couples in their eighties what their secret is. They may be too shy to tell you. If you're single, why do you think the websites for mature singles are humming? Orgasms are good for us. If a partner isn't an option, buy a toy or two online. In moderation, it really isn't self-*abuse*, whatever you've been told. It is the best stress-reliever in nature.

Over time certain things become so much part of our lives that we are a little taken aback if we can't do them. We are creatures of habit, and exercise is a very good habit to build into your life. This is as good a point as any to touch on the bad habits.

Bad habits

I'm not the boss of you, and unless you've lived in a bubble up to now you're already getting defensive. Yours aren't the only ones listed. Guaranteed.

Negativity is an insidious habit and hard to break. Your friend gets a good job in the city, you tell her the commute will be a killer. Your neighbour puts in beautiful fitted carpets, you tell her that colour will be a devil to keep clean. So-and-so has booked a holiday abroad, and you say the climate is terrible that time of year and the crime rate in the area is a real problem. A new restaurant is overpriced and the food wasn't very good. A newcomer to the area seems a little too enthusiastic to be genuine. A suggested way of solving a problem is unlikely to help. You aren't going to bother to try this, that, or the next thing, because what's the point? You won't enjoy it. You think you are being realistic, but what you doing is sucking the enjoyment out of life. A hard habit to break.

Your smartphone is making you miss out on real life! We started this book in a cafe, people-watching. Even on holiday tourists sit in pavement cafes in some of the loveliest places in the world, all their attention riveted on their electronic umbilical cords. Couples who sit together, lost not in each other but in their toys – for that matter, any social event which turns into people showing each other their wretched phones. *Definitely* a habit to break.

<u>Smoking, drinking, drugs</u> – and this is at the level of bad habit, not full-blown addiction. If you have to stop on the way to work to buy a drink, if your hands shake to the point of being useless if you didn't take your drug of choice, if you grope for your cigarettes when the alarm clock goes off in the morning, you are way beyond bad habit. Habits, by definition, can be relearned. Addiction takes outside help.

The first step to reducing or removing bad habits is to divorce them from the rest of your life. Make smoking time just for smoking – stop what you're doing and go outside (even at home, where you don't have to). No writing or reading, don't even take your coffee or drink. Remove smoking from your normal routine and your cigarette count will not only drop, if you do want to quit at some point it will be a lot easier. Same goes for the "mild" drugs – we're talking bad habits here, not addiction, smoking a joint not shooting up! Mild they may be but don't let them become part of your routine. Drinking, don't keep alcohol at home, spritz your wine when you're out, make every other drink a non-alcoholic soda, drink slowly. If you've finished your drink before your host has finished topping everyone up, that's a warning sign, no matter how well you hold your liquor.

In fact I'd define the line where a habit is crossing into addiction as the point where you *can't* do without it. I guess all dependence comes back to that same addiction test - if you are panicky at the prospect of going without, if your mood changes noticeably, if your peers comment, even jokingly, on your consumption, you have a problem.

Bad habits, on the other hand, *can* be unlearned and you *can* do it.

In purely self-destructive terms, the eating habits of binging, snacking, and junk food addiction are oddly, more of a problem. Smoking, drinking, and drugs, are lifestyle choices but we do have to eat. A lot of junk food is laden with additives designed to make us crave more, and more – how *dare* retailers so cold-bloodedly manipulate us for their profit? Sometimes there's no option but giving up your worst addiction altogether, because moderation isn't an option. For most of us the occasional craving is for something sweet, often late at night, and once you've opened it you have to finish it ... a slice of sugared toast is a better alternative. Sliced bread in the freezer, sugar in the pantry, easy enough to make, not so delicious you'll keep going, and enough to stop random wild temptations to drive to all-night supermarkets.

Diet hacks

Try to teach a contemporary a thing or two about food? When I'm not even a qualified nutritionist? Aye, that'll be right.

You already know a healthy varied diet with lots of seasonal fresh food, especially organic fresh food, contains everything you actually need. Our body stores what it needs and discards the rest so taking a ton of expensive additives on top of a good diet is really just producing high-quality pee. However, the key phrase there was *healthy and varied*, and how many of us really do that? Especially if we are living alone, cooking for one is *such* a bore.

Don't make excuses, make changes.

It is much easier to make a large batch of something which will keep for several days. One example, hybrid coleslaw with added ham, cheese, cherry tomatoes, eaten with a thick slice of good quality bread and butter. Another - big casseroles and curries and freezing extra portions in bags (which are ideally moulded to fit into a suitable saucepan. Handy!) You can keep a batch semi-permanently on the go, or at worst in the freezer, and it is all healthy stuff.

The advantage of the big batch is that food reverts to being fuel, not the highlight of your day. You also never feel you are being rationed, and the odd result is that you are likely to eat less, because you'll take a small serving, and go back if you want more. You often forget to go back.

Some dieticians advocate eating regularly, whether hungry or not. Some more relaxed types say you should never force yourself to eat – if you aren't feeling hungry, don't dutifully eat your usual size meal. If you're hungry later, have a snack. A healthy one, of course. The world won't end.

Eat real food rather than replacements, wherever possible. Humans evolved over millennia to efficiently interact with the flora and fauna which were naturally available. It will take a while longer before we can truly metabolize alternatives stiff with additives, preservatives, chemicals and artificial nutrients. That also means raw sugar is better than refined sugar. Refined sugar is better than chemical sweeteners. Butter is better than margarine. Although there are experts out there who'd disagree, cut down your sugar and butter intake rather than switching.

Don't economize on grocery shopping – buy the best you can afford. There's an old saying we tend to forget nowadays; every dollar spent on the table is a dollar less at the doctor.

Buy organic wherever possible. Even organic foods are not 100% natural but you probably don't have time yourself to grow everything you want to eat. Anyway, picking off bugs by hand makes you suddenly understand why organic farmers had to find a human-friendly solution.

Avoid fad diets, especially starvation ones: the older you get, the more likely they will actually damage you. Food is fuel, and your appetite, if you stop mucking about with it, decreases naturally as you get older. Starving yourself is counter-productive.

You probably *are* eating more than you need to, out of habit. The simplest weightloss hack of all – dish up your normal serving, then put half back in the warmer drawer. Eat slowly, chew well, and thoroughly, Lucille Ball said she chewed everything thirty-five times. That's challenging with soft foods but even the attempt slows eating down dramatically. Don't do anything else while you are eating. Okay, if you aren't alone you're allowed to talk! No computer, no TV, not even a book. Concentrating on what you are eating is surprisingly filling. After an hour, if you're still peckish, get the other half of your meal. Don't feel obliged to finish it. If there's a lot left put it into a container in the fridge, and if it was something like spaghetti Bolognaise or curry, it will of course taste even better when re-heated.

Ever loved something that threw your system into a loop as you got older? Some of those reactions will have faded again. Try small amounts. Could be good news.

Drink a lot of water: filtered water is better than bottled water and more environmentally friendly. Green tea, red tea, white tea, chamomile tea, seem to be safe options anytime. Coffee and red wine are fine in moderation.

Seasoning is fine (spices like turmeric and cinnamon are actively good for you) and if you haven't already, switch to coarse salt in a grinder rather than table salt. It's strong, so you'll use less of it.

Avoid over-processed food. That includes some things considered healthy—two examples being soy sauce and commercial fruit juice. The more processed a food is, the fewer nutrients remain, and the more chemicals and preservatives have been added. Chemicals and preservatives are good for keeping food from going bad, but they are not good nutrition.

Anything marked low fat is likely to be higher in sugar, or vice versa, and over-processed.

Any packaged snack with a shelf-life of months, no matter how beguiling the low calorie count is, should be avoided. Your body hasn't evolved yet to cope. It will store the entire snack as fat and send up a message saying *hey, still waiting for food here. Feed me.*

Mealtimes

The nutritionists tell us that within an hour or two of waking, your body needs fuel, and keeping it properly fuelled all day will put a spring in your step and improve your health overall. In Scotland they say the best breakfast for slow-burning energy, especially in cold weather, is oatmeal porridge. That's all very well, but whether it is served with cream and a drizzle of honey or with salt, making it properly takes time. The quick add-boiling-water alternatives are over-processed. Getting up an hour earlier to make a good breakfast does not appeal to all.

Quickest option, if you keep cold meat, hardboiled eggs or cheese on hand, is a protein breakfast. Fruit is not the best start to the day, as it spikes your blood sugar. Two slices of toast are better than a chemical-crammed breakfast-bar.

Snacking during the day is best when you stop what you are doing to eat it slowly and savour it, even if you are at your desk.

Supper should ideally be at *least* two hours before bedtime and not too heavy - your digestion is on a 24-hour clock but don't overload it.

Shopping – heavy on basic ingredients rather than pre-made meals. Protein is good for hair, skin, health, digestion but yes, expensive if you're buying organic chicken, beef and pork. Oily fish and veg high in protein will help. Dairy, all good, Greek yoghurt is healthier than most others, add your own colours and fruit to natural yoghurt. Cheap honey is sugar digested by bees. Proper honey is very expensive.

Make your own salad dressings, even mayonnaise (easy in a food processor) with olive oil and balsamic vinegar to make them actively good for you.

Pasta should be kept to a minimum and never overcook it -the softer it gets, the more fattening it becomes. Most pasta now is made from commercially-grown genetically-modified wheat which was developed to build rapid bulk in livestock, so dial it back unless, of course, you are looking for rapid bulk.

Additives

Add only what you might not be getting enough of. Dislike oily fish? Codliver oil capsules will keep your joints click-free. That sort of thing. Some of the really beneficial additives, in the right quantities, can become lethal when you take too much. Calcium, for example, can have some fairly nasty creeping side-effects - gas, constipation, confusion, kidney stones and muscle weakness, for starters. If you are experiencing any of those symptoms and are taking tablets, cut back. Way, way back.

In fact that applies to all additives. Don't put your uncomfortable symptoms down to the creeping years, and *never* push up the dosage to compensate. Check everything you are taking for side-effects on-line, not on the package, and don't trust the advice of a supplier making money from selling stuff to you. Too much of a good thing can kill you.

That comment about cutting back, by the way, can even apply to prescribed medication, although obviously speak to your doctor before making changes. Over a period of time all medications build up in your system. Sometimes switching to an equivalent is necessary, at least for a while. Not every busy doctor remembers that.

Getting *really* basic – healthy bowel movement is the result of healthy diet and a properly-functioning digestive system. If you start alternating frequently between constipation and the opposite, without any obvious dietary triggers, ask your doctor for a DIY (and post in) test kit. Bowel-screening kits are routine in many countries after the age of fifty five. Polyps becoming increasingly common as we get older, cause havoc, and are easily removed, but shouldn't be left. There's a fashion for using a support to lift your feet, so your position is closer to the original crouch on the ground of our distant ancestors. It is supposed to be fantastic for constipation and generally good for effortless passage (probably for giving birth too, who knows).

Who dares, wins

Is living quietly to a ripe old age with a comfortable sum in the bank to leave to the next generation your definition of a truly happy and successful life? It is for most - and yet a truly surprising number of people are changing their lives completely at this age. Mortgages have been paid off, offspring are independent, there could be an inheritance, or early retirement with a nice pay-out. There's more disposable cash than there was, a lessening of the chains of responsibility, and with it comes restlessness, because life has rarely been the adventure we had hoped it would be.

Few of us, for starters, had the career we once hoped to have. Parents, circumstances, necessity, obligations and even debt, dictated the direction of our working lives from early on. It's been said no-one lies on their deathbed wishing they'd spent more time at the office. Well, deathbeds aren't the time to plan a change. The time could be now.

The changes can be taking up a sport you always wanted to try, make the decision to travel and explore, learn a musical instrument, take painting lessons or try something creative. They *can* be huge - giving up work to turn a hobby into a source of income, or selling up to start a new life abroad, taking one last giant gamble for a last chance at the life we had wanted. A few are spectacularly successful. Many aren't, in material terms. As often as not, standard of living takes a drop, the gamble fails to perform as brilliantly as hoped. Life in a cage is safe. Life on the outside isn't.

So should you, or shouldn't you?

The first rule in gambling is never to bet more than you can afford to lose. You could play safe, set a budget and be prepared to lose your stake - then it won't be crippling if you do, and all the sweeter if you succeed. Happiness is never guaranteed, but the pursuit of it is rarely wasted time. If you are lucky, completing the dreams checklist is just a case of making arrangements, liquidising a few assets, and putting your Indian summer energy to work. Sometimes, though, your life has to be turned upside down and inside out and sensible has to be tossed out with the trash.

Some real life examples: the guy who sold up everything to buy a business on a tropical island. He works harder, at sixty, than ever in his life before. He's invigorated, purposeful, completely happy. The woman who followed a new man to another country, to restart life at fifty-eight. The relationship failed, the house she had bought at the height of a housing boom couldn't be sold at any price, and she had to stay put. Four years later she said it was the best card life ever forced on her. One couple sold up and bought a luxury camper when he retired, planning easy unstressed travel for the rest of their lives. Three years later his health crashed. They sold the camper and bought a much smaller house than the one they had sold, with easy access to the hospital facilities he now needs. Failed dream, yes. Wasted years? Oh no. They are emphatic about that. I said in the introduction I'd changed my whole life too. Would I have been better off if I had never gambled? Yes, financially secure, but it wasn't a happy life. No regrets.

If you have a dream to follow, be aware they rarely play out as planned. And yet - we get one life. At the end of it, what will have counted for most - the challenge we met, or the safety we banked? What price happiness?

Quick fixes / pick-me-ups

This is an excessively girly chapter, all about looks and especially achieving a dramatic change in appearance. If you have a special event coming up, or want to kick-start feeling good, there are quite a few things that will give you a boost. This section assumes an event, because sometimes we need to be jolted out of the comfort of *sometime* into **now.**

A haircut. Consider adding highlights to frame your face, and a layered cut to add bounce. If you have a lovely hairdresser who treats you as a human being, all the better. One of the infuriating things about getting older is their tendency to present any client over fifty with nice granny waves. Do *not* permit that to happen. Discuss options with your stylist - you may decide to head towards a completely different style which needs your hair to grow out a bit, and they can start the process with a trim which will start the new shape in the right direction. If you colour your hair and have used the same colour for years, time for a change. Dramatic blonde, or the very dark colours, are hard to carry off as you get a bit older - as a general rule, softer colour is more flattering. (Blokes, you too. A flat colour with no hint of grey isn't fooling anyone.)

A manicure improves the appearance of your hands immediately. Nicely shaped nails, whether buffed or painted, give you a tiny lift every time you notice them.

Whiten your teeth. Your pharmacy will have a paint-on quick-fix. It feels oddly grainy, and your smile won't be blinding, but there will be a definite, confidence-building, difference. (Be warned, red wine and beetroot could turn your smile pink, read the label.) There are also products sold in gum-trays you can fit onto your teeth which make you drool like an old bulldog during the process, but the results are effective for several days.

Use eye-whitening eye drops. The eye bath is better, long-term, but this is quick fix time.

Vaseline is your quick fix friend. Soak your hands in warm water for ten minutes, then gently smooth on Vaseline to trap the moisture for longer. Use a tiny dab of it to sleek your eyebrows, and leave a faint highlighting shine on your brow bones. You can even smooth a fine layer on your cheekbones and lips, if you don't wear makeup. Don't look sticky, just very slightly shining with health.

You use a moist sponge for applying **foundation**, right? Even the best on the market need that, or they can look caked on. The advantage of a light coating of foundation on mature skin is that it evens out your skin colour, covers the fine lines, and smooths out your general appearance. There are some especially for rewinding time, which do a really good job on the fine lines. If you're trying a new one, experiment a couple of days before The Event. You won't look dramatically younger, but you will look well-rested and good. Light-reflecting primer is the autumn rose's friend. Go easy on the eyeshadow. The idea is to look as if you aren't wearing makeup, or at the most have applied a dash of lippy. Add lip-gloss.

Get your eyebrows professionally shaped, and keep them tidy thereafter. Don't go overboard - the plucked and painted look is a bit freaky, but shaggy brows only suit elderly gents who have the nostril and ear hair to balance them out.

Get fitted for a new **bra**, for an instant improvement to your silhouette. All department stores carry body-shaping **underwear**, take advice and try on different types. The most effective will be the most uncomfortable, though. No good achieving an hourglass figure but looking miserable. Moderation.

If this super-quick makeover is for a **special event**, avoid salt, which can make you retain water, and the gassier vegetables, which can make you bloat, for a couple of days beforehand. You'll probably also see any bags under your eyes improve, too, they're buggers for storing salt.

If you have a few weeks in hand and this is a major event, you can push the boat out with some cosmetic non-surgical procedures. I did, for my daughter's wedding, because I had been following my own advice and had lost quite a lot of weight. Downside, the new creases from mouth to chin made me look like a cross between Deputy Dawg and Charlie McCarthy. The pretty name given to these is marionette creases. Aw, that's sweet. NOT. There are lots of non-surgical cosmetic options available, once you go looking, but dermal fillers, injections to plump out the creases, did seem to be what was needed.

It stung, and stung, and STUNG. Redness and swelling continued for about twelve hours, and the bruising lasted about two weeks, earning me a lot of startled glances. I did look well-rested at the wedding, though, and the confidence boost was worth every penny.

Ageing gracefully

The reality, which is why I wrote this book for those of us who need the facts put in **bold** and <u>underlined</u>, is that there comes a time when you no longer make a strong first impression. Invisible happens. The world, and the workplace, is filled with people younger than you, vigorously getting on with their lives. Don't fight back with garish makeup, overbright clothes and demanding attention, but the absolute opposite, fading into beige, isn't the autumn rose option. Dolly Parton said of her looks, "it takes a lot of money to look this cheap," and it does take a fair amount of work to look as if you're aging effortlessly and gracefully. So - why bother? Who's looking?

Same reason you tidy your home for visitors. Same reason you use the good plates for guests. No one *cares* that you aren't a perfect 10, you know. Why should they? It only matters to you. But you *will* notice people are reacting slightly differently. That's a boost.

Taking care of yourself, walking, eating, exercising, makes you more positive, builds a happy outlook. Those lines round your mouth can make you look sullen even when you think you look expressionless. Smile rather than look neutral, be alert and open, listen as well as talk.

DO NOT FEAR. Fear is so desperately crippling, and the world seems determined to whip us into a permanent state of it. Much of what you fear will never happen, not to you personally. Most of the stuff that does happen is unexpected anyway. When and if it does, deal with it. Fear offers us nothing.

DO NOT REGRET. The past is unchanging. Nothing you can do can change what happened. Take the lesson from it, yes: those who ignore history are fated to repeat it. But do not regret. Nothing that happened to you, if you survived it, can break you, unless you let it. Even grief should become a celebration of what was, not a grinding weight.

GO WHERE YOU WANT TO GO – to visit, even to live – what's holding you back? Time? Money? Fear? If you really want to go somewhere, *carpe diem*, seize the day. Do it.

EAT WHAT YOU WANT. You may need to eat it in smaller quantities, sure. But life is short. You don't really want to cram your face with garbage, but you don't want a life lived on prunes and bran, denial and occasional binging. Treat yourself with quality.

SEIZE EVERY CHANCE TO SEE YOUR FRIENDS. No-brainer. We seasoned mature mellow people can let life distract us, put things off to tomorrow and tomorrow and tomorrow. If the chance comes up to see a favourite person, no, it is not too far. It is not too much trouble. The chance may not come up tomorrow. Do it.

SMILE AND LAUGH. Have you smiled today? Laughed? Or are you reading this thinking that's all well and good but life isn't always funny. No, it isn't. A genuine laugh, though, is like a shot of vitamins, the effect is extraordinary. Smile, now, at the book. Smile at people. Go hunting through YouTube to find good comedians, nostalgic songs which bring back happy times, favourite film clips - we need the habit of smiling. The laughter will follow. It feels *wonderful.*

DON'T EXPECT APPROVAL. Part of this journey is realising we are still youthful at heart, but we probably don't have all the time in the world after all, and there are a lot of things on that to-do list that haven't yet been ticked off. Don't expect support or encouragement, just go do them. Take no notice of what others say about you and even less notice of what they might be thinking. Let them talk, because no matter who you are and what you do, *someone* will disapprove. We get one life.

Splurge occasionally. Buy the best you can afford for those you love, but include yourself: treat yourself to something you've always wanted.

BEING ALONE IS FINE. BEING LONELY, NOT SO MUCH. If you're alone, you don't have to be. There are hundreds, thousands, of people who would jump at the chance of meeting others in the same boat. It's a given that life leaves lumps, bumps, scars, and baggage and no-one you are going to meet will be free of those, any more than you are. Life also brings resilience, humour, and experience and people you meet will have those too. A stranger is just a friend you haven't met yet? Well, maybe not quite that glib. But by reaching out, you will make friends: do it. Have realistic expectations, and have fun. Don't sit at home and get old before your time. At the very least, look at *meetup* for your area, you could be astonished at how much is going on around you.

As for being single and dating, second time round, the idea of meeting someone romantically can seem alarming. It is. If you go that route, you will meet some very odd people, have some alarming encounters, you will feel your blood fizz and your heart creak, but you will definitely feel alive and stimulated. For some bizarre reason, Society looks askance at older people dating, flirting, having affairs. Goodness me, why? Don't we all want affection, shared laughter, even passion, for the rest of our lives?

Take hold today. *Carpe diem*, and step into the sunshine. Enjoy it! And enjoy every day from now on, to the end of your life. Make it a life to remember with pride, maybe with a breathless laugh or two.

Life is a learning curve and we are learning all the time.

About the author

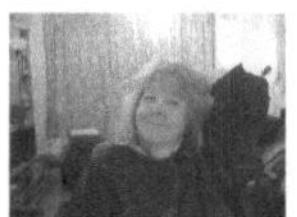

I know I have sounded like a know-it-all, and to be completely honest with you, I have no idea whether I'm getting it generally right or completely wrong. I do know I'm having fun, and that this age is proving unlike any other. I'm braver, bolder, my own person in a way I have never been. No-one's appendage – not someone's daughter, wife, mother, or colleague, I am *ME*.

I wrote this book at sixty, (when the above photo was taken) and said at the time "this gift may last only months. It may be years. I am in my third year of second adolescence and it could all end tomorrow. Right now, though, I am having the best time of my life."

The reason I wrote it at all was that I nearly missed this whole Indian summer thing, nearly wasted it feeling restless and dissatisfied but too brainwashed to do anything about it. There's a persistent perception that we go straight from menopause to old, and we *so* don't. The direct and indirect results included meeting an awful lot of people who are out there celebrating their autumn sunshine, including many, seven years later, now well into their seventies. They remain a constant inspiration.

Back when the unexpected sun first came out I didn't set out to write a series of novels that celebrate this stage of our lives, but it did turn out that way. I write also – mainly – as EJ Lamprey. In the first *Grasshopper Lawns* whodunit, Edge was fifty-eight but could have been any age between fifty-five and seventy-five, her life was so sedate. By the tenth book, the four friends were living life to the full. They can be whoever they want, just so long as their health and vigour holds out, and they are ageless. Just like us. I get annoyed when I'm told that when I get to that age, I will see things differently. I *am* that age. I have younger friends who are already starting to fret and worry, and think themselves old. I have older friends confidently leading the way through the Indian summer and back into the autumn and the crisp bracing winter beyond. The most I will concede is that none of us have solved actual murders.

I haven't lived on another planet either, but as Joanna Lamprey I wrote the *Place* books, celebrating a future where new planets are initially colonised by those over fifty, bringing their experience and vigour to completely new levels. That's not the storyline, just a background fact.

EJ Lamprey and Joanna Lamprey books are, mainly, cosies. The Clarissa novels are more about being a mature single. There's some overlap on that celebration of being rich in years. After *Second Rainbow* a reviewer remarked that she'd expected a more factual guide to being a mature single, so I wrote one (*Looking for Mr Will-Do-Nicely*) and then, why not, this one. The full list of books follows. There's an excerpt from *Rainbow* after that.

Other books available

DO-OVER (thriller)
THE PASSING OF MRS PARKER WOODBURN (novella)
PIDGIN SPANISH (non-fiction)
Children's novella
THE KIDNAP CAPER

Writing as Joanna Lamprey
NO PLACE LIKE PLACE – The Talian Project (book 1)
NO PLACE LIKE PLACE – The Missionaries (book 2)
TIME AFTER TIME (short stories and novella)

Writing as Clarissa Rodgers-Briskleigh
A SECOND RAINBOW
THE MONEY HONEY
Non-fiction
ON PERFECTING YOUR INDIAN SUMMER
LOOKING FOR MR WILL-DO-NICELY

A Second Rainbow

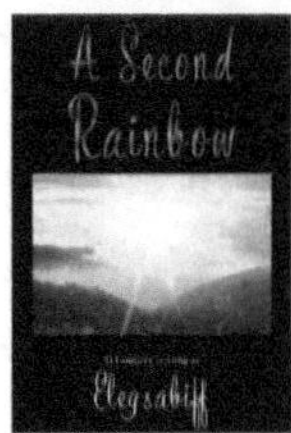

The road to the City of Emeralds is paved with yellow brick. (L Frank Baum, The Wonderful Wizard of Oz)

(Chapter Two)

'I've found a man!' Emma leaned triumphantly against the kitchen worktop, and moved along obediently as Dorothy mildly shooed her. It was October, and rain lashed at the windows, but the kitchen, newly repainted, was bright and cheerful. 'He's perfect! Recently single, *nice*-looking rather than good-looking, in a good job, and not living too close or too far away, about an hour away. If he's a disaster at least there's no chance of bumping into him in the shops!'

'Recently single?' Dorothy glanced up, concerned. 'How old is he?'

'Old enough.' Emma picked up the cup of tea Dorothy had made for her, looked expectantly over the rim at her mother's puzzled face, and burst out laughing. 'Not for me, Mum! For you!'

'Oh, well, good. You gave me a bit of a shock, I thought you and Charlie were getting on very well at the moment. I really don't want a man, you know. That's behind me now.' She picked up the tray to lead the way into the charming little drawing room, then creased her forehead. 'What on earth do you mean, you *found* him?'

Emma started to explain, almost gabbling in her haste as Dorothy looked more and more disapproving. It was, she said artfully, as though Gran herself had been guiding her. There'd been an article on the growing number of baby boomer singles, and the flood of singles websites catering for the rush. Emma noticed a particular website because of its name – *Yellow Brick Road*. If that wasn't a sign . . . So she had taken matters into her own hands. She had joined the website as *DorothyRainbow*, posted a couple of photos, fielded the first approaches, disapprovingly deleted the unsuitable and couldn't resist corresponding with *ScareCrowe*, who signed himself more conventionally as Simon. He wanted to meet for dinner on Friday so she thought it was time Dorothy took her rightful place in this promising encounter. She opened her laptop on the rosewood desk and danced her fingers over the keys as she logged into the website.

Dorothy had to admit Simon was pleasant-looking, with a shock of unruly blond hair, a lumpy nose broken in his football past, and a disarming grin which crinkled his eyes attractively in the close-up photo. In his other photo he had obviously kept his athletic physique, a bit softened around his middle, and his messages had been increasingly lengthy and chatty. Emma's replies, in Dorothy's name, had been what she might have written herself, apart from the terrifying *'yes I would love to meet up'*.

'I *can't.*' She was appalled. 'I never even thought of dating again and I'm certainly not ready for it. What on earth would I say to a total stranger? What if he wants to kiss me at the end of the evening? I'd probably throw up with fright! Anyway, he wouldn't, he's younger than me. Men of that age don't date *older* women.'

Emma was as decisive as her father. 'Rubbish. He knows your age, and he knows what you look like. I know *exactly* what you're going to wear, that new suit you bought, and I have a blouse that's perfect for it which you're going to borrow because your own blouses are a little frumpy. Sorry, but they are. I even worked out how you're going to do your hair, and I've already booked your hair appointment for Friday afternoon. I'm going with you, because I know exactly how they have to do it.'

She looked briefly frustrated that she couldn't cut and style hair herself, then shrugged it off.

'He's tall enough for you to wear heels, and believe me that took some finding because at least half the men who have written were shorter than you. It's a great disadvantage, you being taller than the average woman.'

As Dorothy opened her mouth she added sternly, 'Mum, this is non-negotiable. You *are* going to start dating, because you will probably live another thirty years and you'll be bored rigid if you spend them on your own. I'm not saying Simon is the one, I don't think he is, he's a little too bland and amenable and you *are* used to being told what to do. He's nicely unthreatening. Think of him as your first interview, a learning curve to get you back in the market, okay? I promise you can pick your own guy for the next date.'

(Chapter Three)

*As for the Scarecrow, having no brain he walked straight ahead and
so stepped in the holes and fell on the hard bricks. (L Frank Baum,
The Wonderful Wizard of Oz)*

Simon's straw-coloured hair had obviously been rigorously flattened
for their dinner, and equally obviously had a mind of its own, which
Dorothy rather liked. He was like his photographs, and had looked
reassuringly pleased by the sight of her when Emma dropped her off
at the restaurant with some final stern words of advice.

'You look drop-dead gorgeous, and if his messages are anything
to go by he's a non-stop talker. You don't have to do a thing except
nod, smile, and if he gets out of line, you nip off to the loo, send me a
message, and I'll collect you ten minutes later. Otherwise I'll be here
for you at ten-thirty.'

Dorothy had nodded meekly, her artlessly-casual chignon an un-
familiar weight on her head, and asked with a rebellious flicker of
mischief, 'How do I let you know if I want to go home with him?'
She had the satisfaction of seeing Emma startled and got out the car
smiling to herself with a last wave at her suddenly-doubtful daughter.

'Oh, the name;' He laughed, slightly embarrassed. 'My surname *is*
Crowe, so I was Scarecrow all through school. Scared all the birds
away, my mates said. Just call me Simon.' He poured wine for her,

then for himself, and met her eyes candidly. 'I'll be honest, my wife's leaving knocked a lot of the stuffing out of me. I must be a bit thick, I didn't see it coming at all. She took off with a friend of mine – well, I already told you that. I miss him.'

She laughed obligingly at the old joke, then shrugged. 'I know what you mean, I didn't see mine coming either. She's been his assistant for years but I never thought there would be anything like that. She's not really even the standard predatory blonde type. She was married when she started working for him, I have no idea whether she started after him when she got divorced, or even whether she got divorced because of him.'

Obedient to Emma's orders to keep the conversation in his court, she added politely, 'How did your kids take it?'

'Oh, teenagers are teenagers, they probably haven't noticed yet.' He shrugged ruefully, then bent forward earnestly. 'If your husband's secretary wasn't gorgeous, he needs his sight checked. You *are*. I couldn't believe it when you walked in here looking even better than your profile on the *Road*. Good-looking sane women aren't exactly a feature on singles websites.'

'Maybe I'm not sane?' she suggested, and realised she was starting to enjoy herself. Flattery hadn't played much of a role in her life and Simon's attention, and his involuntary glances down the low neck of Emma's borrowed blouse, was warming her even more than the slightly glib compliments. By the second bottle of wine they were relaxing and laughing together and she felt an unexpected stab of disappointment when she saw Emma appear in the doorway. Three hours *already*?

'I have to go, my lift's arrived,' she said regretfully and his smile slipped instantly.

'Your daughter? Oh well, I'm looking forward to meeting her. Dorothy, I haven't enjoyed an evening so much in years. When can I see more of you?'

'More of me, or see me again?' she asked recklessly, and blushed deeply even as she said it. He blinked, recovered, and covered her hand with his own.

'Both. As soon as possible.'

'What was the blushing about?' Emma asked inquisitively as they drove home and Dorothy grinned involuntarily.

'You win. He was nice,' she answered instead. 'He has a dinner tomorrow that he can't get out of but we're meeting on Sunday afternoon. He's taking me to a pub he knows which does great meals and then coffee and brandy around a roaring fire. He said we'll need it after the walk we're doing in the afternoon. And he's bringing his dog.'

'Meeting the dog, wow, big step. Mum, you'll be careful, won't you? There are some funny men on singles websites, and sometimes the nicer they seem, the dodgier they turn out to be. I'm not surprised he's fallen for you but I'd be really worried if you got too keen on him.'

'You said it yourself, he's my learning curve.' Dorothy was dismissive but in the darkness of the car she smiled secretly to herself. Simon, she decided, if he was willing, was going to help her learn a great deal.

Dorothy's affair with Simon ends, and she goes on to meet the Tin Man and the Cowardly Lion, but although this is a book about dating and the extremely odd men and women involved in the second-time-round world it is as much about life, love, laughter, betrayal and friendships. A must-read, even if only as a cautionary tale, for anyone considering entering what really is a different world –